Withdrawn

Bicton College of Agriculture
636.08979   28163
Learning Resource Centre

Quick Reference Guide to Veterinary Surgical Kits

Senior commissioning editor: Mary Seager
Development editor: Caroline Savage
Production controller: Anthony Read
Desk editor: Jackie Holding
Cover design: Alan Studholme

Quick Reference Guide to Veterinary Surgical Kits

Carole Bowden DipAVN (Surgical) VN and
Jo Masters VN

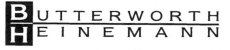

BUTTERWORTH
HEINEMANN

OXFORD AUCKLAND BOSTON JOHANNESBURG MELBOURNE NEW DELHI

Butterworth-Heinemann
Linacre House, Jordan Hill, Oxford OX2 8DP
225 Wildwood Avenue, Woburn, MA 01801-2041
A division of Reed Educational and Professional Publishing Ltd

A member of the Reed Elsevier plc group

First published 2001

© Reed Educational and Professional Publishing Ltd 2001

All rights reserved. No part of this publication may be reproduced in
any material form (including photocopying or storing in any medium by
electronic means and whether or not transiently or incidentally to some
other use of this publication) without the written permission of the
copyright holder except in accordance with the provisions of the Copyright,
Designs and Patents Act 1988 or under the terms of a licence issued by the
Copyright Licensing Agency Ltd, 90 Tottenham Court Road, London,
England W1P 0LP. Applications for the copyright holder's written
permission to reproduce any part of this publication should be addressed
to the publishers

British Library Cataloguing in Publication Data
Bowden, Carole
Quick reference guide to veterinary surgical kits
1. Veterinary surgery – Equipment and supplies
I. Title II. Masters, Joanne
636'.089'79178

ISBN 0 7506 4958 5

Typeset by BC Typesetting, Keynsham, Bristol BS31 1NZ
Printed and bound in Great Britain by MPG Books Ltd, Bodmin, Cornwall

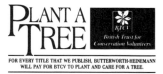

FOR EVERY TITLE THAT WE PUBLISH, BUTTERWORTH-HEINEMANN
WILL PAY FOR BTCV TO PLANT AND CARE FOR A TREE.

Contents

Introduction   vii

1 **Surgical terminology**   1

2 **General surgical equipment**   3
   Instruments   3
   Suture materials   7
   Drapes and disposables   12
   Theatre requirements   17

3 **Surgical preparation**   21
   Preparation of surgical equipment   21
   Preparation of the surgical environment   23
   Preparation of surgical personnel   24
   Preparation of the patient   26
   Health and safety   28

4 **Surgical procedures**   29
   Abdominal surgery   29
   Orthopaedic surgery   43
   Perineal surgery   65
   Miscellaneous surgical procedures   71

5 **Self-assessment**   86

Selected reading   92

Index   93

Introduction

The aim of this book is to provide an easy reference point for those veterinary staff involved in theatre preparation. It is not intended to be used as a textbook, more as a handy guide which can be kept in the preparation room for easy referral.

This guide will be invaluable to both student veterinary nurses preparing for a specific procedure for the first time and to veterinary staff anticipating an unfamiliar surgical procedure.

Each section is designed to cover the basic range of equipment necessary for routine surgical procedures; however, flexibility for individual preferences should be assumed.

The authors and publishers would like to gratefully acknowledge the support and help which they have received from Arnold's Veterinary Product Ltd in the production of this book.

1
Surgical terminology

Surgical veterinary terms consist of two parts:

(i) THE PREFIX – or first syllable of the word; often used to describe the anatomy in question. For example:

hyster – uterus
cyst – bladder
enter – intestines
osteo – bone

(ii) THE SUFFIX – or last syllable(s) of the word; often used to describe the procedure. Surgical suffixes include:

OTOMY – surgically forming a temporary opening, e.g.
Laparotomy – forming a temporary opening into the abdomen
Cystotomy – forming a temporary opening into the bladder
Enterotomy – forming a temporary opening into the intestines
Hysterotomy – forming a temporary opening into the uterus

OSTOMY – surgically forming a permanent opening, e.g.
Urethrostomy – forming a permanent opening into the urethra
Gastrostomy – forming a permanent opening into the stomach
Tracheostomy – forming a permanent opening into the trachea

ECTOMY – surgically removing a structure (or part of), e.g.
Ovariohysterectomy – removal of the ovaries and uterus
Orchidectomy – removal of the testes
Splenectomy – removal of the spleen

CENTESIS – removal (aspiration) of fluid from a body cavity, e.g.
Paracentesis – aspiration of fluid from the abdomen
Thoracocentesis – aspiration of fluid from the thorax
Cystocentesis – aspiration of urine from the bladder

OSCOPY – examination of a structure with a specific instrument, e.g.
Endoscopy – examination with an endoscope

PLASTY – surgical shaping or formation, e.g.
Arthoplasty – formation of a new joint

Terminology is also used to describe both the surgical approach to be used and the possible risks of the procedure due to wound contamination.

Surgical approaches

Examples include:

- **Midline** – incision through the linea alba
- **Paramedian** – incision to one side of the linea alba
- **Parapreputial** – incision to one side of the prepuce
- **Paracostal** – incision just caudal to and parallel with the last rib

Wound classification

- **Clean** – a surgical incision made in aseptic conditions that does not enter the respiratory, alimentary or urogenital tracts (e.g. orchidectomy)
- **Clean–contaminated** – a surgical incision made in aseptic conditions which does enter the respiratory, alimentary or urogenital tracts (e.g. enterotomy)
- **Contaminated** – a surgical incision or fresh traumatic wound with a major break in aseptic technique (e.g. aural ablation)
- **Infected** – a traumatic wound which is more than 6 hours old or surgery involving perforated viscera in the abdomen

2
General surgical equipment

Instruments

There is a wide range of instruments available for all surgical procedures. A good knowledge of the basic instrument classifications will aid in identification and correct selection for use within specific kits.

Individual preferences and the type of surgery to be undertaken need to be borne in mind when selecting instrument kits.

Standard instruments

Scalpel blade handle
This instrument aids with the control and action of the scalpel blade when attached, allowing for precision incisions to be made.

Scalpel blades
These come in a variety of shapes and sizes. The commonly used sizes are 10, 11 and 15 (see Figure 2.1).

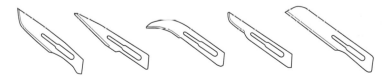

Figure 2.1. Types of scalpel blade.

Dissecting forceps
These come in a wide range from simple Bendover forceps, Treves rat-tooth forceps to Adson Brown forceps. Their main aim is to hold tissues. Those with plain ends are used for holding delicate, friable tissue, whereas the 'rat-tooth' variety can be used to hold dense connective tissues.

Scissors
Mayo scissors are the most frequently used scissors in veterinary surgery. They can be used for simple cutting techniques or blunt dissection. Where fine delicate dissection is required, Metzenbaum scissors can be employed.

Artery forceps
These forceps are used for haemostasis by clamping blood vessels prior to placement of a ligature. They may be curved or flat with transverse striations within the jaws. Names of those commonly used are Spencer Wells, Halstead mosquito and Dunhill.

Tissue forceps
These instruments are designed to grasp tissue causing minimal trauma. Allis tissue forceps, Lanes tissue forceps and Babcocks are examples of these.

Towel clips
These are designed to attach the surgical drapes to the patient. Two commonly used clips are Backhaus and Grays cross-action towel clips.

Needle holders
As the title suggests, these instruments hold the suture needles. They can also have a scissor action as well to avoid the use of two instruments during suturing. Those providing needle holders and stitch scissors are Gillies and Olsen Hegar. Those providing just needle holders are McPhails, Bruce Clarke and Mayo Hegar.

Retractors
Retractors are designed to hold tissue apart in order to improve visualization of the surgical site and internal organs. They may be self-retaining or hand held. Gelpi, Travers and West are examples of self-retaining retractors, whereas Lagenbeck and Malleable are examples of hand-held retractors. For deep abdominal or thoracic surgery, Balfour or Gossett self-retaining retractors can be employed.

Visceral clamps
Clamps are used for the occlusion of visceral lumen, the most common being Doyen clamps (bowel clamps) designed to facilitate the occlusion of the intestinal lumen.

Ophthalmic instruments

Instruments used for ophthalmic procedures are basically smaller variations on standard instruments as stated above. Those employed for specialist ophthalmic surgery are beyond the scope of this book.

Dental instruments

Hand scalers
These instruments remove calculus from the tooth surface. Sub-gingival scalers have one sharp edge and one moulded edge, and are designed to remove calculus from the gingival sulcus. Supra-gingival scalers have two sharps edges designed to remove calculus from the gingival margin to the tip of the tooth.

Elevators
These instruments are designed to loosen the tooth root as an aid to extractions. They come in a variety of sizes and angles.

Extraction forceps
These forceps act as pliers by gripping the tooth and aiding in extraction of the tooth from the jaw. They come in a variety of shapes and sizes.

Dental probes
These are designed to measure the depth of the gingival sulcus and also detect any entry into the pulp cavity due to trauma.

Orthopaedic instruments

Bone-holding forceps
These instruments are designed to hold and grasp bone fragments. They can be designed to hold single or twin fragments and can be hand held or self-retaining.

Bone cutters and rongeurs
Rongeurs are used for nibbling small pieces of bone or cartilage. Bone cutters such as Listons are designed to cut larger pieces of bone. An orthopaedic hacksaw and blade can also be used to cut bone. Chisels, osteotomes, gouges and curettes are often employed to cut, remove or shape bone or cartilage. A Gigli wire and handles can also be employed in some cases to saw through bone.

Bone rasps
These instruments help to reshape bone or cartilage by removing any sharp edges. An example is the Putti rasp.

Retractors
Standard retractors such as Gelpi and Travers can be employed; in addition to these, the hand-held Hohmann retractor is frequently used.

Wire cutters and twisters
These are employed to twist wire evenly and tightly followed by cutting it neatly.

Drills and drill bits
Drills may be hand driven or battery driven. A wide range of drill bits is available for all orthopaedic procedures (see Figure 2.2).

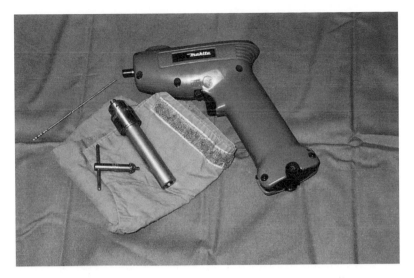

Figure 2.2. Electric hand drill and bits.

Orthopaedic fracture fixation

Several implants are available to provide stabilization of the fracture site. For simplicity they have been listed as follows:

- Intramedullary pins – Steinemann and rush pins
- Bone plates – Venables, Sherman, ASIF and decompression (DCP, ASIF)
- Screws – self-tapping or tapped screws, Sherman, ASIF, cortical and cancellous
- External fixators – pins, connecting bars and clamps
- Wire – Cerclage stainless steel or Kirschner wire

Suture materials

Several different suture materials can be employed in one surgical procedure (Figure 2.3). In order to understand the reasons for use, you first need to understand their basic properties and classifications.

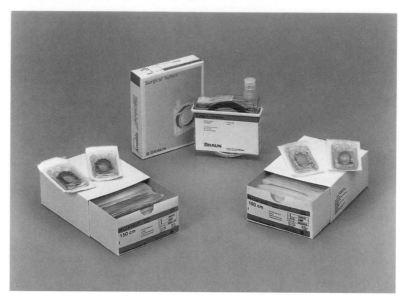

Figure 2.3. Range of suture materials.

Ideal characteristics of suture materials

- High tensile strength – high breaking strength
- Good knot security – knot should hold securely and tie easily
- Minimal tissue reaction – biologically inert
- Good handling properties – easy to handle with minimal memory of its packing configuration
- Non-capillary – should not encourage wicking of fluid
- Absolute biodegradability – predictable rate of absorption
- Readily available and economic

Classification of sutures

- Multifilament – several strands joined together
- Monofilament – one single strand of material

Table 2.1. Natural and synthetic sutures

Suture	Natural	Synthetic	Absorption rate (average)	Absorption method
Chromic catgut	✓		14–21 days	Phagocytosis
Polyglycolic acid		✓	14–21 days	Hydrolysis
Polyglactin 910		✓	14–21 days	Hydrolysis
Polydioxanone		✓	90 days	Hydrolysis

Absorbable

These materials degrade within the tissue and lose their tensile strength over approximately 60 days depending on the individual properties. They can be subdivided into natural and synthetic sutures (see Table 2.1).

Non-absorbable

These sutures maintain their tensile strength for longer than 60 days and are used where prolonged mechanical support is required (see Tables 2.2 and 2.3).

Table 2.2. Non-absorbable sutures

Suture	Natural	Synthetic
Silk	✓	
Multifilament nylon		✓
Monofilament nylon		✓
Stainless steel		✓

Table 2.3. Suture material selection

Area	Selection
Skin	Monofilment nylon or metal staples
Subcutis	Synthetic absorbable
Muscle	Synthetic absorbable
Viscera	Synthetic absorbable
Tendon	Non-absorbable or high tensile strength non absorbable

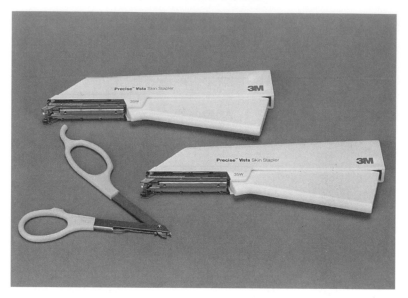

Figure 2.4. Skin stapler.

Alternatives to suture materials

Tissue glue or skin staples (see Figure 2.4).

Suture needles

Eyed needles/traumatic needles
These type of needles require threading of the suture material and therefore cause trauma to tissue at the eye of the needle due to the increase in size/lumen (see Figure 2.5).

Atraumatic needles
These needles have the suture material attached directly to the needle (swaged on), therefore avoiding trauma to the tissue as they have an equal size lumen.

Round-bodied needles
These are designed to separate tissue rather than cut through. They tend to be used on delicate tissue such as viscera.

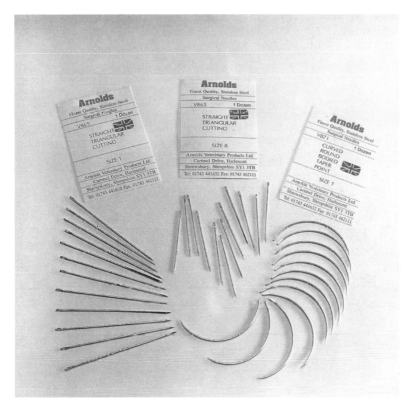

Figure 2.5. Range of suture needles.

Cutting needles
These are used whenever dense tissue is to be sutured. The triangular cutting edge permits easy passage through this tissue. These needles are mainly used in the skin. Needles come in a variety of shapes and their use depends on the area to be sutured:

● Half curved
● Half circle
● Straight

Drapes and disposables

Gowns and Drapes for surgical procedures may be disposable or non-disposable and it will be at the discretion of the Practice as to what is used (see Figure 2.6 and Table 2.4).

Swabs

● Swabs will be either prepacked and sterilized or packed within the veterinary practice to individual needs/ requirements

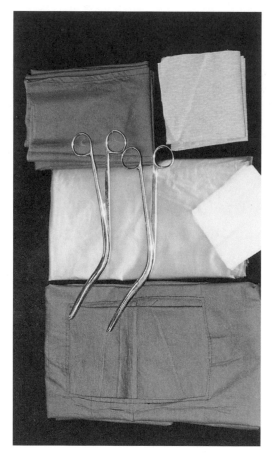

Figure 2.6. Range of draping materials.

Table 2.4. Gowns and drapes

Classification	Advantage	Disadvantage
Disposable	Less laundry Usually water repellent Pre-sterilized Consistent quality	Expensive Non-conforming Large stock needed
Non-disposable	Cheaper Conformable Smaller stocks required	Porous Time consuming Quality deteriorates with time and use

- It is essential that all packs are clearly marked with the total number of swabs
- Standard size cotton swabs (10 cm × 10 cm) are usually employed for routine procedures
- Large laparotomy swabs can be employed with the more involved procedures, and where haemorrhage and lavage is involved
- Ideally the swabs will have a radio-opaque strip within them for easy detection by radiography if required

Disposables

A selection of the following sterile equipment should be readily available should they be needed for surgical procedures (Figures 2.7 and 2.8).

- Intravenous catheters
- Intravenous fluid replacement bags and infusion sets
- Fluid for abdominal lavage
- Spare surgical drapes and gloves
- Urinary catheters
- Spare swabs
- Suction tips
- Sample collection pots
- Surgical drains (Figure 2.9)

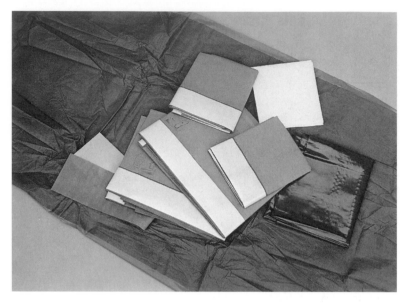

Figure 2.7. Selection of disposables: I.

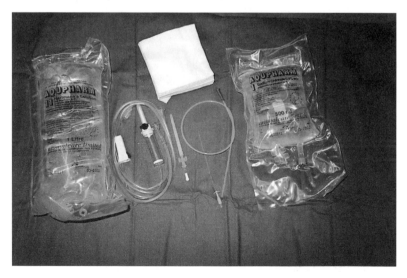

Figure 2.8. Selection of disposables: II.

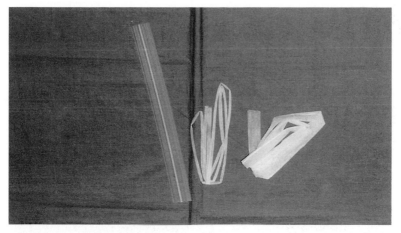

Figure 2.9. Surgical drains.

Miscellaneous equipment

There will be other pieces of equipment that will be used within the theatre on occasions for specific procedures. It is essential that you familiarize yourself with reference to their whereabouts, preparation and use.

Diathermy unit

Diathermy is a technique which either cuts or coagulates tissues. High-frequency electrical currents produce heat at the site of application of the needles or forceps (see Figure 2.10). Diathermy is used to:

- Control haemorrhage
- Reduce the number of ligatures
- Decrease surgical time

It is essential to use an 'earthing' plate between the patient and work surface when using this piece of equipment.

Cryosurgical unit

Cryosurgery destroys living tissue by application of extreme cold. Its aim is to kill cells in a designated area while producing

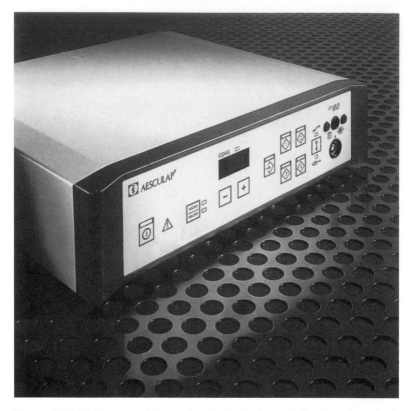

Figure 2.10. Diathermy unit (reproduced with kind permission from Aesculap).

minimal effect on the surrounding tissues. The unit is filled with liquid nitrogen. A rapid freeze via a probe or fine jet is followed by a slow thaw and then the cycle is repeated as necessary (see Figure 2.11).

Endoscopes
Endoscopes are extremely expensive pieces of equipment that require careful handling. They are used to visualize body cavities or hollow organs, usually via the thoracic or gastrointestinal tract (see Figure 2.12). There are two types of endoscope available:

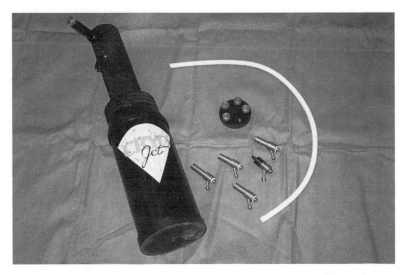

Figure 2.11. Cryo unit.

- Rigid – useful for bronchial and oesophageal
- Flexible (as fibre optic or video) – used for gastrointestinal

Suction unit
A suction unit can be used for aspiration of fluid and suction of fluids and blood during surgery. There are many types available and a size suitable for the Practice requirements will normally be chosen (Figure 2.13). Separate sterile suction tips can be made available for the surgeon or nurse to attach to the main apparatus for use during surgery.

Theatre requirements

See Figure 2.14.

Ideal properties

- The operating theatre should be sited so as to avoid and discourage unnecessary movement of personnel and patients

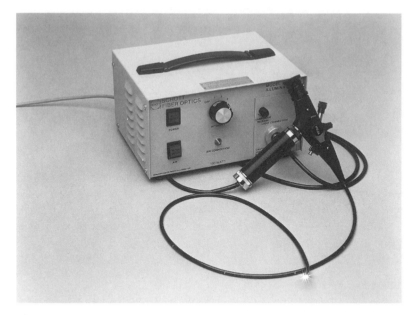

Figure 2.12. Endoscope.

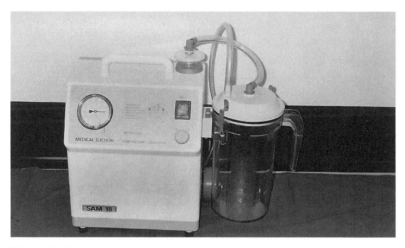

Figure 2.13. Suction unit.

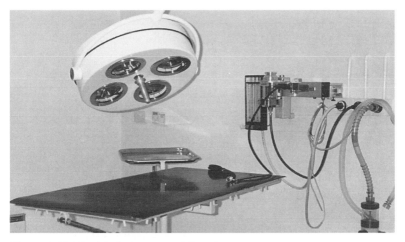

Figure 2.14. Ideal theatre – essential equipment.

- There should be a clear separation of sterile, clean and dirty areas
- There should be no cupboards or shelves within the theatre
- Essential equipment only – anaesthetic machine, operating table, drip stand, X-ray viewer, Mayo table, instrument trolley and kick bowl (Figure 2.15)
- Other equipment must be kept to a minimum
- Walls, floors and ceilings should be easily washable
- Floors should be non-slip and antistatic
- Good lighting is essential
- Heating should be controlled at a constant temperature of between 15 and 20°C
- A scavenger system for anaesthetic gases must be provided
- Ventilation and air conditioning systems are desirable
- A supply of electrical sockets recessed in the wall
- Dry wipe board for recording swabs, blood loss, etc.
- A clock

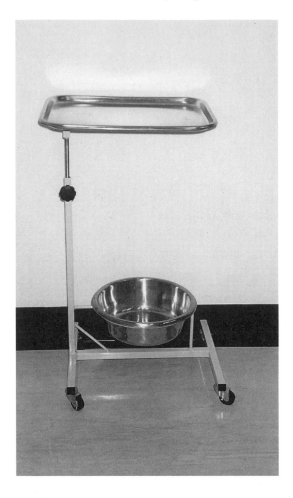

Figure 2.15. Instrument trolley and kick bowl combination.

3
Surgical preparation

Good preparation techniques are essential to the success of the surgical procedure. Thought should be given to the preparation of the equipment to be utilized, the theatre environment, the personnel involved and the patient to be operated on. Health and safety considerations should also be taken into account.

Thought also needs to be given to the organization of the operating list to minimize the risk of contamination from both the surgical team and the environment. Procedures should be organized into 'clean', 'clean–contaminated', 'contaminated' and 'infected' categories and dealt with in that order (refer to p. 2).

Preparation of surgical equipment

All surgical equipment should be regularly maintained to keep it in good working order. Look for signs of damage such as faulty cables, burned out bulbs, ratchets not working, cracks in plastic casing, possible contamination problems, etc. Examples of surgical equipment which should be maintained in this way are:

- **Anaesthetic equipment** (including monitors, circuits, endotracheal tubes, etc.) – check gas levels, leaking valves, perished rubber, exhausted soda lime, cracks and punctures in tubing, electrical faults, etc.
- **Ancillary equipment** (diathermy, suction, cryo, drills, dental scalers, heat pads, etc.) – check performance prior to surgery

- **Theatre equipment** (table, instrument trolley, lights, etc.) – ensure are clean and working properly
- **Preparation equipment** (clippers, razors) – check blades are in good working order
- **Sterilization equipment** (ultrasonic cleaners, autoclaves, etc.) – regular checks on the performance of your sterilizer are crucial

Instrumentation

Follow some basic rules:

- Maintain instruments in dry conditions or they will discolour and rust
- All instruments should be cleaned as soon as possible after use and not be allowed to dry – soaking in COLD water is recommended if cleaning is not to be carried out immediately after use
- When using ultrasonic cleaners, ensure you are using the correct chemical made up to the dilution directed
- Abrasives should not be used – this will roughen the surface leading to pitting, discoloration and rust
- Instruments should not be soaked in chemical solutions for long periods, and should be thoroughly rinsed and dried before use
- Lubricants should be used periodically to prevent joints becoming stiff
- Purified or distilled water should be used in the autoclave – mains water can leave deposits both in the autoclave and on the instruments – costly repairs and replacements
- All new instruments should be thoroughly cleaned, lubricated and sterilized before use
- Always handle instruments carefully to prevent damage from dropping, etc.

Disposables

Have supplies of suture equipment to hand as well as an extra sterile instrument pack to use if contamination occurs.

Ensure that extra packs of sterile swabs are easily available should they be required during surgery.

Preparation of the surgical environment

Thought should be given to the preparation of both your theatre and preparation areas. This should include:

- **Vacuuming** – This is preferable to sweeping the surgical area, which increases the amount of airborne microbes; however, a separate vacuum should be kept for this purpose rather than using one that is utilized around the whole Practice. Ideally a theatre should have its own wet vacuum or a central vacuum system.
- **Damp dusting** – All surfaces in the surgical area should be damp dusted with a mild disinfectant solution prior to use. Include any anaesthetic equipment and do not forget to dust the top of surgical light fittings. Damp dusting should be carried out one hour before the procedure is scheduled to take place.
- **Washing walls** – All walls should be washed down with a disinfectant solution both before and after a surgical procedure. The ideal method is to start at the top of the wall and work down to discourage microbes from being transported up the wall from the floor. Do not forget to include window sills, skirting boards, extractor fans, etc. Cloths should ideally be either disposable or freshly laundered for each use.
- **Mopping** – Mops can carry many microbes around the Practice and the surgical area should have its own designated mopping equipment. A freshly laundered mop head should be used each time the floor space of the surgical area is cleaned and the disinfectant used should be of an appropriate type for theatre use.
- **Kick bowls and waste receptacles** – These should be lined to prevent contamination and should be emptied either when full or between procedures.

Preparation of surgical personnel

All members of the surgical team should abide by clear preparation rules:

- Personnel hygiene – regular showering/washing of hair, etc.
- Finger nails should be kept short and smooth. Nail polish should not be worn
- All jewellery should be removed
- Long hair should be tied back

Ideally a clean scrub suit (or clean surgical gown), theatre shoes/footcovers, surgical cap and mask should be worn by all personnel entering the theatre area (see Figure 3.1).

Surgical personnel involved in sterile surgical procedures should be wearing theatre clothing before performing a surgical scrub, and donning a sterile gown and gloves.

Surgical scrub

The aim of the scrub routine is to remove micro-organisms from the hands (see Figure 3.2).

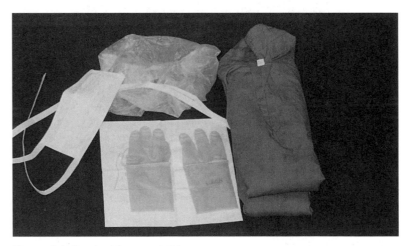

Figure 3.1. Surgical theatre clothing.

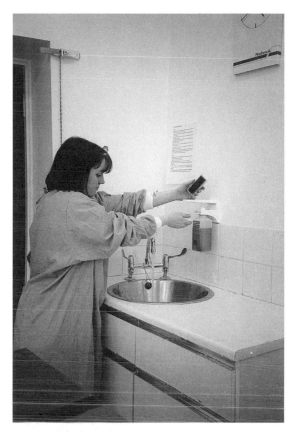

Figure 3.2. Surgical scrub.

Equipment required:

- Sink with elbow controls
- Scrub solution (such as chlorhexidine)
- Sterile scrubbing brush
- Sterile towels
- Sterile gown
- Sterile gloves

A recommended surgical scrubbing procedure should be used which includes scrubbing of individual fingers, palms, backs of hands and forearms using a routine which starts at the tip of the fingers and finishes at the forearms covering all the areas in between. Scrub procedures vary in length of time; a long scrub of 10 minutes may be used at the beginning of the operating list with shorter scrub routines being carried out between procedures.

Sterile towels, preferably one for each hand, should be offered after scrubbing, followed by a surgical gown and, lastly, surgical gloves.

Preparation of the patient

Prior to the anaesthetising and preparation of any surgical patient, verification of its identity, the procedure to be carried out and the patient's history should take place. The existence of a signed consent form should be confirmed (see Figure 3.3).

Equipment required:

● Kidney dish/receptacle – to enable expression of the bladder
● Clippers – surgical preparation blade size A40
● Vacuum cleaner
● Surgical scrub solution (such as povidone/iodine)
● Gauze swabs (or cotton wool swabs)

The sex of the animal should be checked at preparation for reproductive surgery.

Urine may need to be expressed or faecal matter may need to be removed prior to surgery. The surgical area will need to be clipped and the clipped hair vacuumed away.

A surgical scrub routine should be carried out on the operating site using a surgical scrub solution and swabs. This routine should ensure that the solution is in contact with the skin for the required length of time (dependent on solution used) and that the rinsing procedure works from the incision site outwards to prevent contamination.

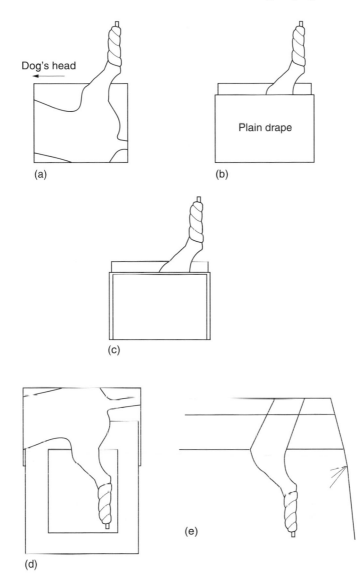

Figure 3.3. Patient preparation.

Health and safety

Health and safety considerations for the surgical team include:

- Faulty equipment – such as frayed electric cables
- Misuse of equipment – overheating, etc.
- Inflammable products – e.g. alcohol-based solutions/diathermy equipment
- Injury from surgical instruments – ensure instruments are used carefully and for the purpose for which they have been designed
- Injury from 'sharps' – ensure all sharps are properly disposed of after use; removal of scalpel blades before surgical instruments are soaked can be forgotten
- Zoonotic diseases – wear gloves when handling all clinical waste

Other health and safety problems can occur from inadequate anaesthetic scavenging and poor ventilation in the theatre.

4
Surgical procedures

Abdominal surgery

Kits within this section are formed from a basic surgical kit that can be used for any laparotomy procedure. Specific kits have been identified for the following procedures:

- Cystotomy
- Enterotomy/enterectomy
- Exploratory laparotomy
- Orchidectomy
- Ovariohysterectomy
- Splenectomy

NB. *Where* clean–contaminated *surgery (e.g. enterotomy, cystotomy) is to be performed, it may be advisable to have a minor surgical kit available in addition to the main kit. This minor kit may be used for closure of the peritoneum and surrounding tissues, therefore eliminating contamination.*

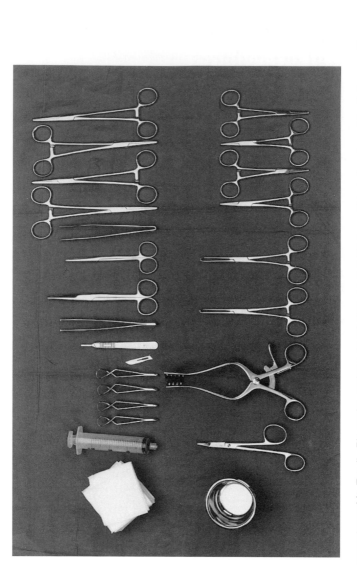

Figure 4.1. Laparotomy kit. Top (L–R): swabs, syringe, towel clips, scalpel blade and blade handle, rat-tooth forceps, Mayo scissors, Metzenbaum scissors, dressing forceps, 4 × large Spencer Wells forceps. Bottom (L–R): galipot, Gillies needle holders, Travers retractors, 2 × Allis tissue forceps, 4 × Spencer Wells forceps.

Laparotomy

A basic surgical kit suitable for laparotomy procedures should contain (Figure 4.1):

- Drapes
- 4 × Towel clips
- Scalpel blade and handle
- Rat-tooth forceps
- Dressing forceps
- Mayo scissors
- Metzenbaum scissors
- 4 × Large Spencer Wells forceps
- 4 × Small Spencer Wells forceps
- 2 × Allis tissue forceps
- Retractors
- Galipot
- Swabs
- Sterile syringe
- Needle holders

Other uses for this kit include:

- Gastrotomy
- Mastectomy
- Multiple tumour removals
- Hernia and rupture repairs
- Repair of ruptured diaphragm

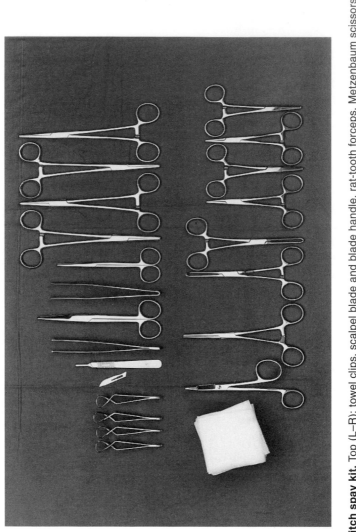

Figure 4.2. Bitch spay kit. Top (L–R): towel clips, scalpel blade and blade handle, rat-tooth forceps, Metzenbaum scissors, dressing forceps, Mayo scissors, 4 × large Spencer Wells forceps. Bottom (L–R): swabs, Gillies needle holders, angiotribes, 2 × Allis tissue forceps, 4 × Spencer Wells forceps.

Ovariohysterectomy (bitch spay)

A bitch spay kit should include (Figure 4.2):

- Drapes
- 4 × Towel clips
- Scalpel blade and handle
- Rat-tooth forceps
- Mayo scissors
- Dressing forceps
- Metzenbaum scissors (*optional*)
- 4 × large Spencer Wells forceps
- 4 × Small Spencer Wells forceps
- Angiotribes (*optional*)
- 2 × Allis tissue forceps
- Swabs
- Needle holders
- Suture materials

Other uses for this kit include:

- Hysterotomy – Caesarean section – clean–contaminated
- Ovariohysterectomy for endometritis (pyometra)

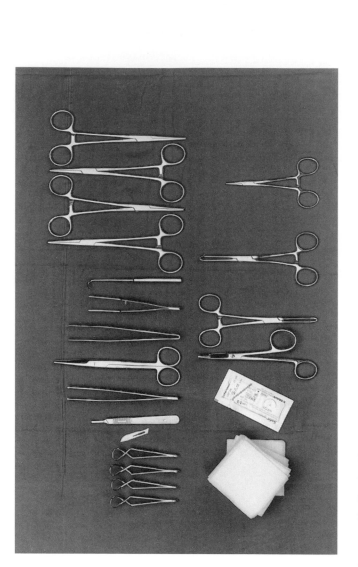

Figure 4.3. Cat spay kit. Top (L–R): towel clips, scalpel blade and blade handle, rat-tooth forceps, Mayo scissors, dressing forceps, spay forceps, spay hook, 4 × Spencer Wells forceps. Bottom (L–R): swabs, suture materials, Gillies needle holders, Allis tissue forceps, mosquito forceps.

Ovariohysterectomy (cat spay)

A cat spay kit should include (Figure 4.3):

- Drape/towel clips
- Scalpel blade and handle
- Rat-tooth forceps
- Mayo scissors
- Dressing forceps
- Spay forceps
- 4 × Spencer Wells forceps
- Needle holders
- Suture material
- Swabs
- Spay hook (*optional*)
- Mosquitos (*optional*)
- Allis tissue forceps (*optional*)

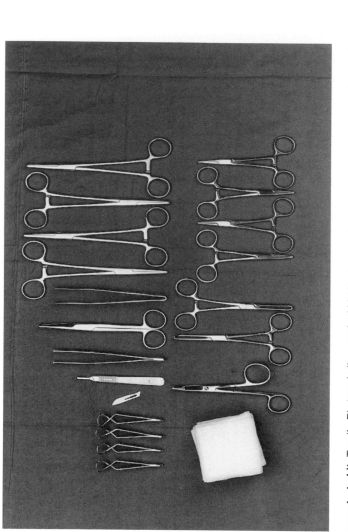

Figure 4.4. Dog castrate kit. Top (L–R): towel clips, scalpel blade and handle, rat-tooth forceps, Mayo scissors, dressing forceps, 4 × large Spencer Wells forceps. Bottom (L–R): swabs, Gillies needle holders, 2 × Allis tissue forceps, 4 × small Spencer Wells forceps.

Orchidectomy (castration)

The castration of a cat requires very little in the way of instrumentation. A scalpel blade, handle and a pair of Spencer Wells forceps should be available (Figure 4.4).

A dog castrate kit should include:

- Drape/towel clips
- Scalpel blade and handle
- Rat-tooth forceps
- Mayo scissors
- Dressing forceps
- 4 × Large Spencer Wells forceps
- 4 × Small Spencer Wells forceps
- 2 × Allis tissue forceps
- Needle holders
- Suture material
- Swabs

Other uses for this kit include:

- Cryptorchidectomy
- Scrotal ablation

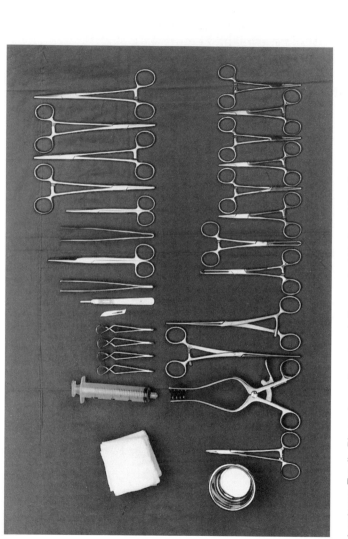

Figure 4.5. Enterotomy. Top (L–R): swabs, syringe, towel clips, scalpel blade and handle, rat-tooth forceps, Mayo scissors, dressing forceps, Metzenbaum scissors, 4 × large Spencer Wells forceps. Bottom (L–R): galipot, Mayo needle holders, Travers retractors, doyen forceps, Allis tissue forceps, 6 × small Spencer Wells forceps.

Enterotomy/enterectomy (opening into/removal of part of the intestines)

This kit would be suitable for surgery of the small or large intestine. A minor surgical kit should be available for closure of the peritoneum (Figure 4.5).

- Drape/towel clips
- Scalpel blade and handle
- Rat-tooth forceps
- Mayo scissors
- Dressing forceps
- Metzenbaum scissors
- 4 × Large Spencer Wells forceps
- 6 × Small Spencer Wells forceps
- 2 × Allis tissue forceps
- 2 × Doyen forceps
- Retractors
- Needle holders
- Suture material
- Swabs
- Galipot
- Syringe

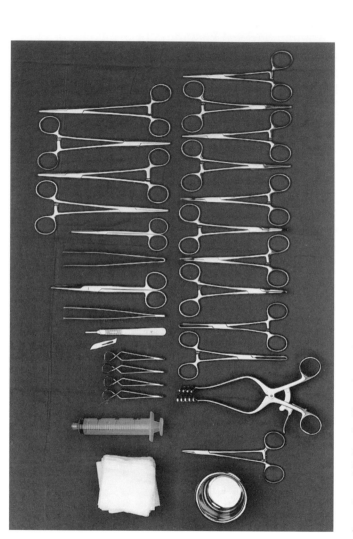

Figure 4.6. Splenectomy kit. Top (L–R): swabs, syringe, towel clips, scalpel blade and handle, rat-tooth forceps, Mayo scissors, dressing forceps, Metzenbaum scissors, 4 × large Spencer Wells forceps. Bottom (L–R): galipot, Mayo needle holders, Travers retractors, 2 × Allis tissue forceps, 8 × Spencer Wells forceps.

Splenectomy (removal of the spleen)

Extra haemostats and swabs are essential requirements for this
procedure (Figure 4.6):

- Drapes/towel clips
- Scalpel blade and handle
- Rat-tooth forceps
- Mayo scissors
- Dressing forceps
- Metzenbaum scissors
- 4 × Large Spencer Wells forceps curved
- 8 × Spencer Wells forceps (curved and straight)
- 2 × Allis tissue forceps
- Retractors
- Needle holders
- Suture material
- Swabs
- Galipot
- Syringe

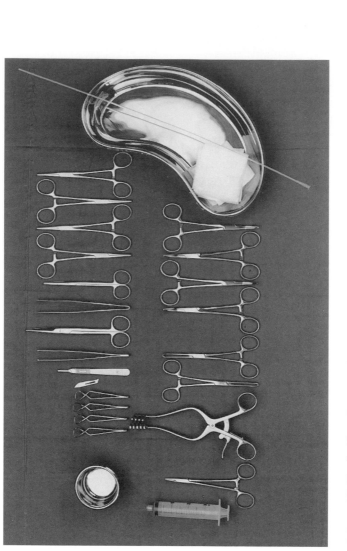

Figure 4.7. Cystotomy kit. Top (L–R): galipot, towel clips, scalpel blade and handle, rat-tooth forceps, Mayo scissors, dressing forceps, Metzenbaum scissors, 4 × Spencer Wells forceps. Bottom (L–R): syringe, Mayo needle holders, Travers retractors, 2 × Allis tissue forceps, 4 × Spencer Wells forceps, kidney dish containing swabs and catheter.

Cystotomy (opening into the bladder)

A means of draining urine from the bladder may be required; therefore the provision of urinary catheters is desirable (Figure 4.7):

- Drapes/towel clips
- Scalpel blade and handle
- Rat-tooth forceps
- Mayo scissors
- Dressing forceps
- Metzenbaum scissors
- 8 × Spencer Wells forceps (curved and straight)
- 2 × Allis tissue forceps
- Retractors
- Needle holders
- Suture material
- Swabs
- Galipot
- Syringe
- Kidney dish
- Catheters as applicable

Orthopaedic surgery

Orthopaedic surgery can encompass a variety of techniques. Each individual case will be different and on occasions several surgical kits may be required for one procedure. It is essential, however, to always provide a general orthopaedic surgical kit. This will provide the basis to build upon for individual requirements.

Orthopaedic kits and instruments have been identified for the following:

- General orthopaedic surgical kit
- General orthopaedic equipment
- Bone-holding forceps
- Rush pins and mallet
- Wiring

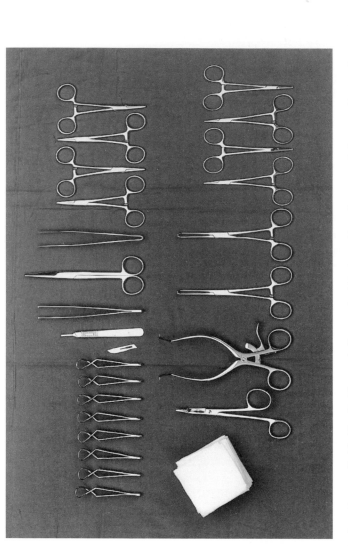

Figure 4.8. Basic orthopaedic kit. Top (L–R): towel clips, scalpel blade and handle, rat-tooth forceps, Mayo scissors, dressing forceps, 4 × small Spencer Wells forceps. Bottom (L–R): swabs, Gillies needle holders, Gelpi retractors, 2 × Allis tissue forceps, 4 × mosquito forceps.

- Plating
- Pinning
- External fixators
- Cruciate ligament repair
- Excision arthroplasty
- Amputation

Basic orthopaedic surgical kit

A basic orthopaedic surgical kit should contain (Figure 4.8):

- Drapes
- 8 × Towel clips
- Scalpel handle and blade
- Rat-tooth forceps
- Dressing forceps
- Mayo scissors
- 4 × Small Spencer Wells forceps
- 4 × Mosquito forceps
- 2 × Allis tissue forceps
- Retractors
- Needle holders
- Suture materials
- Swabs

Additional equipment

Specific orthopaedic equipment.

General orthopaedic equipment

There is a wide range of orthopaedic equipment available for basic handling and cutting/shaping of bone. These instruments can include:

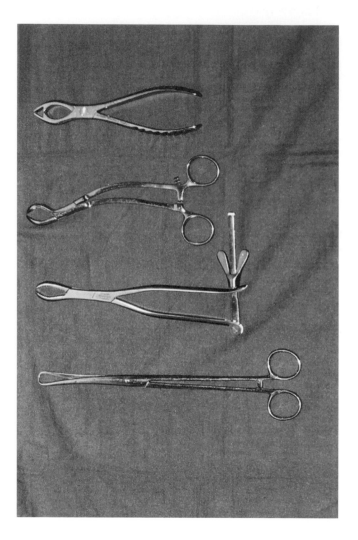

Figure 4.9. Bone-holding forceps.

Cutting/shaping bone and cartilage

- Volkmanns curette
- Periosteal elevators
- Osteotome
- Chisel
- Mallet
- Gouge
- Rongeurs
- Bone cutters
- Putti rasp
- Hacksaw and blade
- Gigli wire and handles
-

Bone-holding forceps (Figure 4.9)

- Single fragment bone holders
- Lowmans bone clamps
- Twin fragment bone holders
- Fergusons bone holders

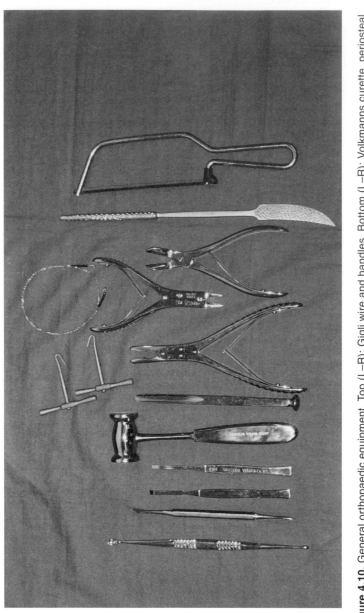

Figure 4.10. General orthopaedic equipment. Top (L–R): Gigli wire and handles. Bottom (L–R): Volkmanns curette, periosteal elevators, osteotome, chisel, mallet, gouge, rongeurs, bone cutters, Putti rasp, hacksaw.

Fracture fixation kits

The method of fracture repair employed will vary between individuals and their predisposing conditions (see Figure 4.10). Some fracture fixation techniques will involve one or two methods and therefore individual kits have been identified as follows.

NB. *Each of the following kits will require a general orthopaedic surgical kit, retractors and bone-holding forceps in addition to those instrument kits stated.*

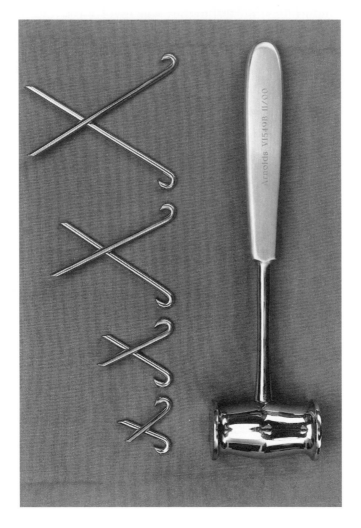

Figure 4.11. Rush pin repair. Rush pins and orthopaedic mallet.

Rush pin fracture repair

Equipment for rush pin application to the epiphyseal area of the bone should contain (Figure 4.11):

- Selection of rush pins
- Orthopaedic mallet

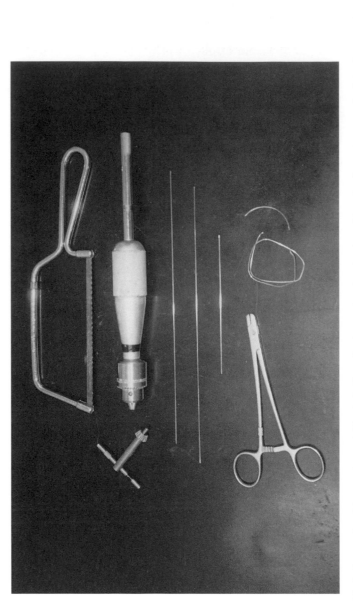

Figure 4.12. Orthopaedic wiring equipment. Top to bottom: hacksaw, Jacobs chuck and key, k-wires, sismeys wire introducer and twisters, wire cutters, Mayo needle, wire suture

Orthopaedic wiring equipment

Essential equipment for basic wiring techniques should contain (Figure 4.12):

- Selection of Kirschner wires
- Jacobs pin chuck and key
- Hacksaw and blade or pin cutters
- Sismey wire introducer and twisters
- Wire cutters
- Mayo needle
- Wire suture

Uses of this instrumentation include:

- Repair of fractured mandibular symphysis
- Epiphyseal fracture repairs
- Tendon repair

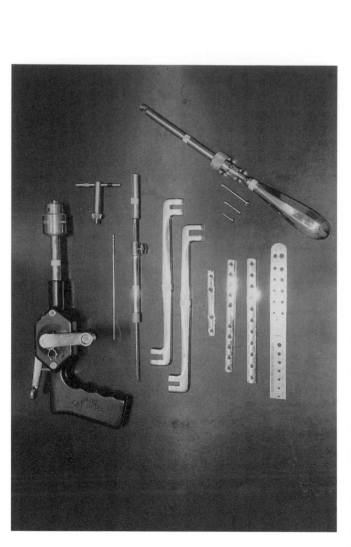

Figure 4.13. Plating equipment. Top to bottom: orthopaedic drill and key, twist drill, depth guage, plate benders, Venables plate, orthopaedic ruler, screws, screwdriver.

Plating equipment

Kits for standard plating techniques should contain (Figure 4.13):

NB. *More specialist plating equipment is available but beyond the scope of this book.*

● Selection of Venables or Sherman plates
● Selection of self-tapping cortical and cancellous screws
● Pair of plate benders
● Orthopaedic screwdriver and shield
● Orthopaedic ruler
● Orthopaedic depth gauge
● Orthopaedic drill, chuck and key, drill bits

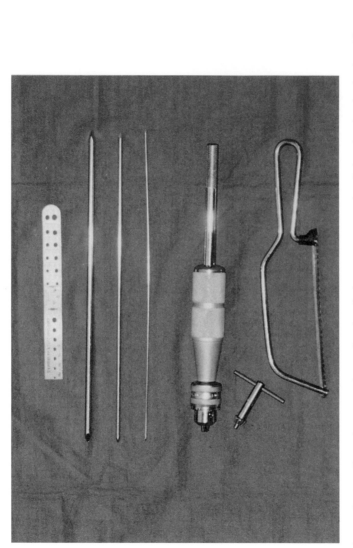

Figure 4.14. Pinning equipment. Top to bottom: orthopaedic ruler, Steinemann trocar pointed pins, Jacobs pin chuck and key, hacksaw.

Pinning equipment

Kits for standard intramedullary pinning procedures should contain (Figure 4.14):

● Selection of Steinemann pins (trocar – pointed both ends)
● Jacobs pin chuck and key
● Orthopaedic ruler and measure
● Pin cutters
● Hacksaw and blade

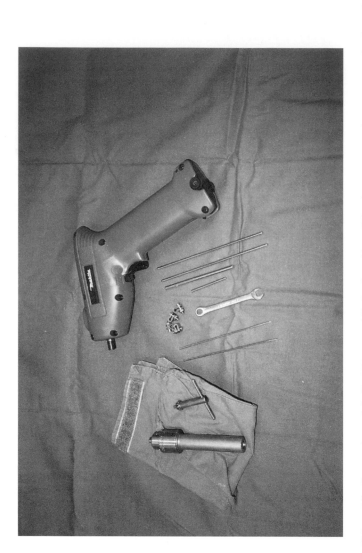

Figure 4.15. External fixation equipment. L–R: drill cover, drill chuck and key, Ellis pins, spanner, clamps, connecting bars, hand drill.

External fixation

Equipment for external fixation procedures may be on occasions used with pinning equipment. A general kit for external fixation should include (Figure 4.15):

- Drill, chuck and key
- Drill bits
- Drill cover
- Selection of Ellis pins (plain and threaded)
- Connecting bars
- Clamps
- Spanner
- Pin cutters

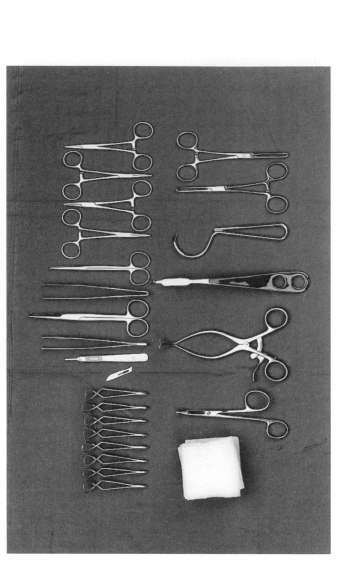

Figure 4.16. Cruciate repair kit. Top (L–R): towel clips, scalpel blade and handle, rat-tooth forceps, Mayo scissors, dressing forceps, Metzenbaum scissors, Spencer Wells forceps. Bottom (L–R): swabs, Gillies needle holders, Gelpi retractors, Hohmann retractor, graft passer, Allis tissue forceps.

Cruciate repair kit

The method of cruciate repair will depend on the individual injury and the surgeon's choice. Equipment for cranial cruciate repair involving the use of a fascia graft for stability of the joint should contain (Figure 4.16):

- Drapes
- 8 × Towel clips
- Scalpel handle and blade
- Mayo scissors
- Treves rat-tooth forceps
- Metzenbaum scissors
- Selection of small artery forceps
- 2 × Allis tissue forceps
- Gelpi retractors
- Hohmann retractors
- Graft passer
- Mayo needle
- Needle holders
- Suture materials
- Swabs

Alternative techniques may require the provision of drill, chuck and key, drill bits, and Putti rasps.
Other uses for this kit include:

- repair of luxating patellas
- trochleaplasty

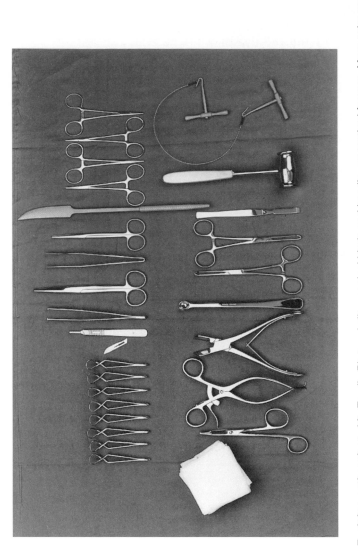

Figure 4.17. Excision anthroplasty kit. Top (L–R): towel clips, scalpel blade and handle, rat toothed forceps, Mayo scissors, dressing forceps, Metzenbaum scissors, putti rasp, Spencer Wells forceps. Bottom (L–R): swabs, Gillies needle holders, Gelpi retractors, bone cutters, teresector, Allis forceps, chisel, mallet, Gigli wire and handles

Excision arthroplasty kit

The size and type of equipment employed in this procedure will depend on the size of the patient. A kit suitable for a cat or small dog should contain (Figure 4.17):

- 8 × Towel clips
- Scalpel handle and blades
- Mayo scissors
- Dressing forceps
- Treves rat-tooth forceps
- Metzenbaum scissors
- 4–6 × Mosquito forceps
- 2 × Allis tissue forceps
- Teresector
- Putti rasp
- Bone cutters
- Gelpi retractors
- Needle holders and stitch scissors

For larger dogs the kit will need to include:

- Orthopaedic chisel
- Orthopaedic mallet, or
- Gigli wire and handles

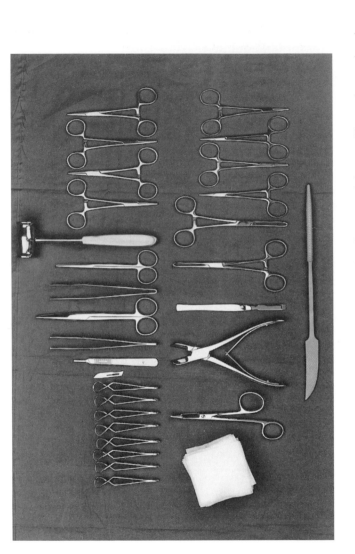

Figure 4.18. Amputation kit. Top (L–R): towel clips, scalpel blade and handle, rat-tooth forceps, Mayo scissors, dressing forceps, Metzenbaum scissors, mallet, Spencer Wells forceps. Bottom (L–R): swabs, Gillies needle holders, bone cutters, chisels, Allis forceps, 4 × mosquito forceps, Putti rasp.

Amputation kit

The size of bone cutters and equipment required for amputation will depend on the site for amputation and the size of the animal. A basic amputation kit should contain (Figure 4.18):

- Drapes
- 8 × Towel clips
- Scalpel handle and blade
- Dressing forceps
- Treves rat-tooth forceps
- Metzenbaum scissors
- 4 × Mosquito forceps
- 4 × Small Spencer Wells forceps
- 2 × Allis tissue forceps
- Bone cutters
- Chisel
- Mallet
- Putti rasp
- Needle holders and stitch scissors

Uses for this kit include:

- Digit amputation
- Limb amputation
- Tail amputation

Perineal surgery

Surgery to this area will be classified as clean–contaminated or contaminated. It is therefore essential to ensure optimum asepsis is achieved in the preparation and procedures in these patients. Double draping of the area is usually employed.

Specific kits have been identified for the following:

- General perineal surgery
- Anal furunculosis
- Anal gland removal
- Urethostomy

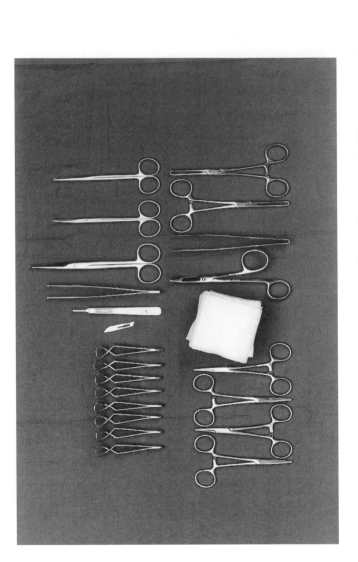

Figure 4.19. General perineal surgery. Top (L–R): towel clips, scalpel blade and handle, rat-tooth forceps Mayo scissors, small curved Metzenbaum scissors, straight Metzenbaum scissors. Bottom (L–R): selection of artery forceps, swabs, Gillies needle holders, dressing forceps, Allis tissue forceps.

General perineal surgical kit

A general perineal surgical kit suitable for all perineal procedures including perineal hernia repair should include (Figure 4.19):

- 8 × Towel clips
- Scalpel handle and blade
- Dressing forceps
- Treves rat-tooth forceps
- Mayo scissors
- Metzenbaum scissors
- 4 × Small Spencer Wells forceps
- 4 × Mosquito forceps
- 2 × Allis tissue forceps
- Needle holders and stitch scissors
- Swabs
- Suture materials

Other uses of this kit include:

- General tumour removal

Anal furunculosis

A basic perineal surgical kit should be used for this procedure plus the following:

- Diathermy unit (unipolar and bipolar)
- Selection of diathermy needles
- Cryosurgery unit
- Selection of probes
- Lubricating jelly

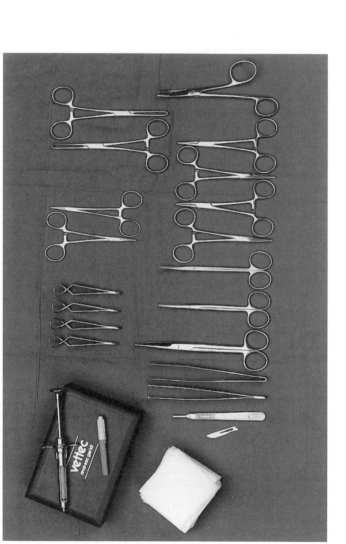

Figure 4.20. Anal gland removal kit. Top (L–R): Vettec kit, towel clips, mosquito forceps, Allis forceps. Bottom (L–R): swabs, scalpel blade and handle, rat-tooth forceps, dressing forceps, Mayo scissors, Metzenbaum scissors (straight and curved), Spencer Wells forceps, Gillies needle holders.

Anal gland removal

Some preparation techniques will need to be employed prior to anal gland removal. Equipment used for this should include:

- Anal gland syringe
- Anal gland needles
- Anal gland wax (pre-heated to body temperature)

The kit should include (Figure 4.20):

- 4 × Towel clips
- Scalpel handle and blade
- Dressing forceps
- Treves rat-tooth forceps
- Mayo scissors straight
- Mayo scissors curved
- Metzenbaum scissors
- 4 × Small Spencer Wells forceps
- 4 × Mosquito forceps
- 2 × Allis tissue forceps
- Needle holders and stitch scissors
- Swabs
- Suture materials

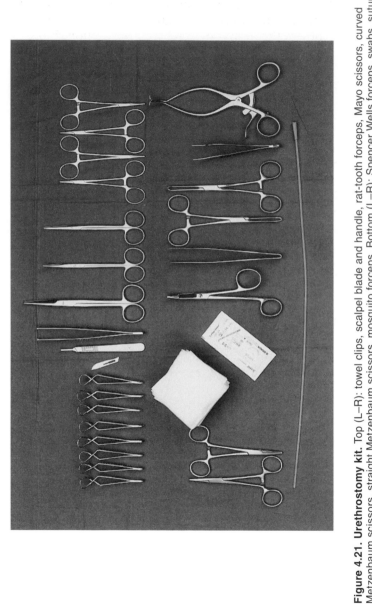

Figure 4.21. Urethrostomy kit. Top (L–R): towel clips, scalpel blade and handle, rat-tooth forceps, Mayo scissors, curved Metzenbaum scissors, straight Metzenbaum scissors, mosquito forceps. Bottom (L–R): Spencer Wells forceps, swabs, suture material, Gillies needle holders, dressing forceps, Allis tissue forceps, Adson Brown forceps, Gelpi retractors, catheter.

Urethrotomy/urethrostomy kits

These kits will follow the same basic principles as for perineal surgery with the addition of urinary catheters. A basic kit suitable for urethrotomy or urethrostomy should include (Figure 4.21):

- 4–8 × Towel clips
- Scalpel blade and handle
- Dressing forceps
- Adson Brown tissue forceps
- Mayo scissors
- Metzenbaum curved scissors
- Metzenbaum straight scissors
- 4 × Mosquito forceps
- 2 × Small Spencer Wells forceps
- 2 × Allis tissue forceps
- Gelpi retractors
- Needle holders and stitch scissors

Miscellaneous surgical procedures

This section includes some of the more generalized surgical techniques. Kits have been identified for:

- Aural surgery
- Ophthalmic surgery
- Thyroidectomy
- Biopsy
- Basic suturing
- Dentistry

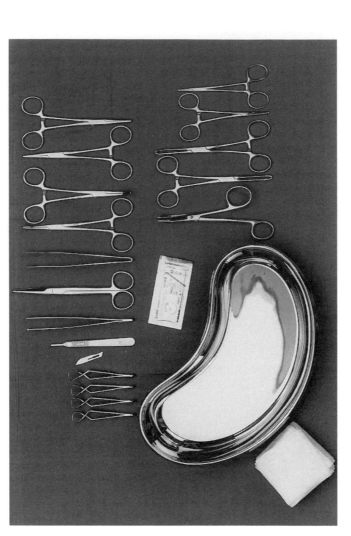

Figure 4.22. Aural surgical kit. Top (L–R): towel clips, scalpel blade and handle, rat-tooth forceps, Mayo scissors, dressing forceps, variety of Spencer Wells forceps. Bottom (L–R): swabs, kidney dish, suture materials, Gillies needle holders, Allis tissue forceps, mosquito forceps.

Aural surgery

Aural surgical procedures include (Figure 4.22):

- Surgery for haematoma
- Repair of split pinnae
- Removal of pinnae/squamous cell carcinoma removal
- Aural resections, such as lateral wall resections and vertical canal ablations

A general aural surgical kit, suitable for all aural surgery should include:

- Drapes
- Towel clips
- Scalpel handle and blade
- Rat-tooth forceps
- Mayo scissors
- Dressing forceps
- Selection of curved and straight Spencer Wells forceps
- 2 × Mosquito forceps
- Allis tissue forceps
- Swabs
- Kidney dish
- Flush
- Needle holder
- Suture material

NB. *Aural surgery is usually either contaminated or infected and should be treated accordingly.*

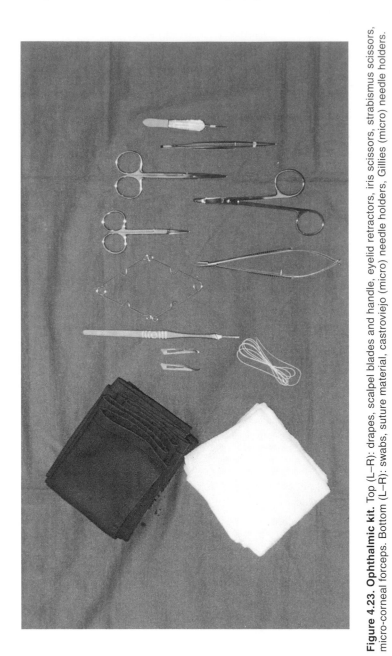

Figure 4.23. Ophthalmic kit. Top (L–R): drapes, scalpel blades and handle, eyelid retractors, iris scissors, strabismus scissors, micro-corneal forceps. Bottom (L–R): swabs, suture material, castroviejo (micro) needle holders, Gillies (micro) needle holders.

Ophthalmic surgery

General ophthalmic surgery includes:

- Entropion/ectropion – correcting inward and outward turning of the eyelid, respectively
- Removal of eyelid tumours
- Distichiasis – removal of supernumerary eyelashes
- Conjunctival flap – third eyelid flap
- Enucleation – removal of the eyeball

A basic ophthalmic kit should include (Figure 4.23):

- Drapes
- Blade and scalpel blade handle
- Eyelid retractors
- Ophthalmic scissors (iris, strabismus or tenotomy)
- Micro corneal forceps
- Micro needle holders
- Suture material
- Swabs

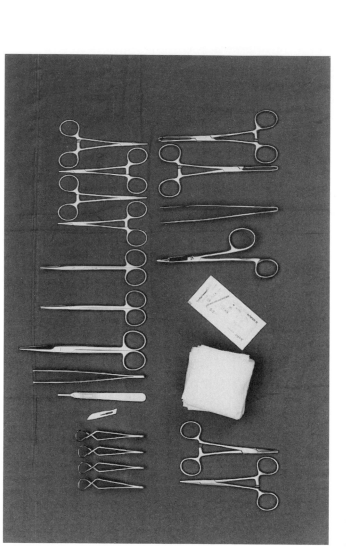

Figure 4.24. Thyroidectomy kit. Top (L–R): towel clips, scalpel blade and handle, rat-tooth forceps, Mayo scissors, Metzenbaum scissors (flat), Metzenbaum scissors (curved), 2 × mosquito forceps. Bottom (L–R): 2 × Spencer Wells forceps, swabs, suture material, Gillies needle holders, dressing forceps, Allis tissue forceps.

Thyroidectomy (removal of the thyroid gland(s))

A thyroidectomy kit should include (Figure 4.24):

- Drapes
- Swabs
- Towel clips
- Scalpel blade handle and blade
- Rat-tooth forceps
- Dressing forceps
- Mayo scissors
- Metzenbaum scissors
- Selection of mosquito and Spencer Wells forceps
- Allis tissue forceps
- Needle holders
- Suture materials

A pathological sample container should be on hand should histopathology be required.

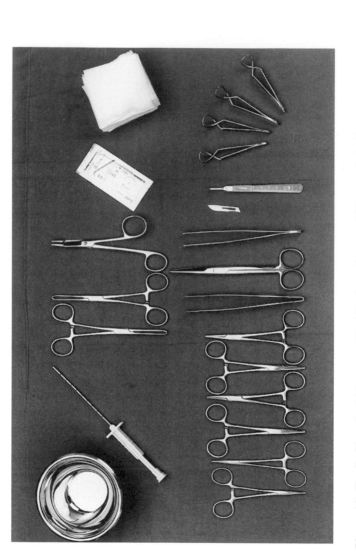

Figure 4.25. Biopsy kit. Top (L–R): galipot, biopsy needle, Allis tissue forceps, Gillies needle holders, suture material, swabs. Bottom (L–R): mosquito forceps, Spencer Wells forceps, dressing forceps, Mayo scissors, rat-tooth forceps, scalpel blade and handle, towel clips.

Biopsy kit

Methods of taking a biopsy include:

- Removing a wedge of tissue
- Using a biopsy punch
- Using a trucut needle

A biopsy kit should include (Figure 4.25):

- Drapes
- Towel clips
- Swabs
- Scalpel blade handle and blade
- Rat-tooth forceps
- Dressing forceps
- Mayo scissors
- 4 × Spencer Wells forceps
- 2 × Mosquito forceps
- Allis tissue forceps
- Suture material
- Needle holders
- Collection receptacle
- Biopsy punch/trucut needle (as desired)

NB. *A pathological sample container should be available for all methods.*

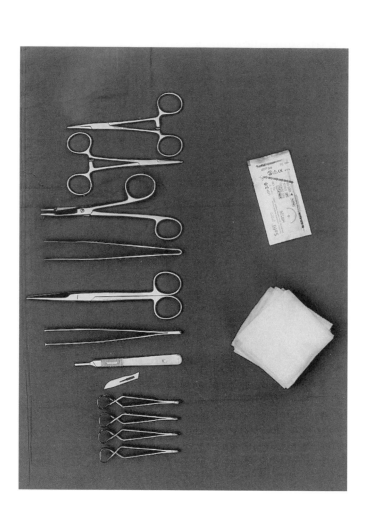

Figure 4.26. Basic suturing kit. Top (L–R): towel clips, scalpel blade and handle, rat-tooth forceps, Mayo scissors, dressing forceps, Gillies needle holders, Spencer Wells forceps. Bottom (L–R): swabs, suture materials.

Basic suturing kit

A basic stitch kit useful for the suturing of minor wounds should include (Figure 4.26):

- Drapes
- Towel clips
- Swabs
- Blade and scalpel blade handle
- Rat-tooth forceps
- Dressing forceps
- Mayo scissors
- 2 × Spencer Wells forceps
- Needle holders
- Suture materials

Other uses of this kit include:

- Minor tumour/cyst removal

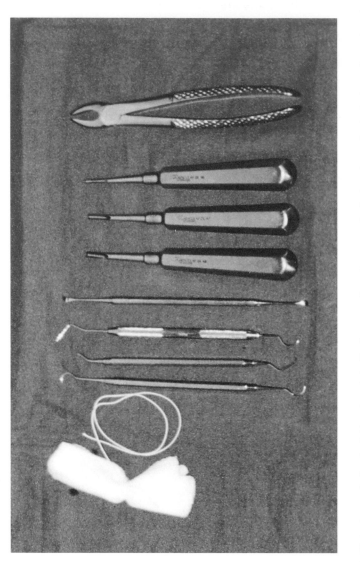

Figure 4.27. Instruments for dental treatment. L–R: pharyngeal swab, supra-gingival scaler, sub-gingival scaler, sub-gingival curette and scaler, sub-gingival scaler, supra-gingival scaler, three dental elevators, extraction forceps.

Dentistry

Dental techniques can be put into two categories:

- Treatment – removal of calculus, dental extractions
- Prophylactic therapies – routine scaling and polishing

Whilst all dentistry can be classed as 'contaminated', every effort should be made to adhere to aseptic technique. Instruments required for dental treatment are shown in Figure 4.27.

Treatment
Instrumentation required for dental treatment will include:

- Retrievable pharyngeal swab
- Supra-gingival curette
- Supra-gingival scaler
- Sub-gingival curette
- Sub-gingival scaler
- Peridontal probe
- A selection of dental elevators
- A selection of extraction forceps
- A dental drill
- Packing material (post-extraction)
- Suture material and instrumentation (post-extraction)

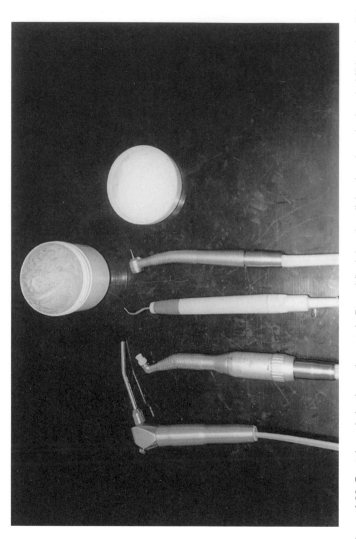

Figure 4.28. Dental prophylactic equipment. L–R: oral flush head, polisher head, scaler head, drill head, polish.

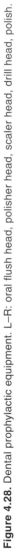

Prophylactic therapies
Instrumentation required for dental prophylactic treatment
includes (Figure 4.28):

- Scaler
- Polisher
- Polish
- Oral flush
- Swabs

Treatment carried out using electrical equipment will be of
superior quality.

NB. *The health and safety implications for dentistry require that
personal protective clothing is worn for all procedures. This
includes:*

- Disposable apron
- Disposable gloves
- Safety spectacles/goggles
- Mask

5
Self-assessment

How well do you score on surgical nursing?

Multiple choice

1. Which ONE of the following is a type of **tissue** forcep?
   (a) Mayo
   (b) Dunhill
   (c) Allis
   (d) Gillies

2. Into which wound classification would an **enterotomy** fit?
   (a) clean
   (b) clean–contaminated
   (c) contaminated
   (d) infected

3. The suffix **centesis** refers to:
   (a) surgical removal
   (b) incision into
   (c) examination
   (d) drainage

4. Which ONE of the following does NOT require sterilization as part of **good aseptic** technique?
   (a) mask
   (b) gloves
   (c) gown
   (d) instruments

5. The effectiveness of a **surgical** scrub depends on:
   (a) time the soap is in contact with the skin
   (b) scrubbing action of the brush
   (c) temperature of the water
   (d) combination of contact time and scrubbing action

6. **Metzenbaum** scissors are MOST suitable for:
   (a) cutting sutures
   (b) soft tissue dissection
   (c) cutting the linear alba
   (d) cutting skin

7. Which ONE of the following is a **non-absorbable** suture material?
   (a) silk
   (b) catgut
   (c) polydioxanone (PDS)
   (d) polyglactin 910 (Vicryl)

8. After what time does **synthetic absorbable** suture lose its tensile strength?
   (a) 120 days
   (b) 30 days
   (c) 60 days
   (d) 10 days

9. The aim of **aseptic** surgical technique is to prevent contamination of the:
   (a) surgical team
   (b) surgical instruments
   (c) surgical drapes
   (d) surgical wound

10. The item of equipment used to **destroy** tissue by the use of extreme cold is a:
    (a) diathermy
    (b) cryosurgery unit
    (c) endoscope
    (d) suction unit

11. The **temperature** in the operating theatre should be around:
    (a) 10–15°C
    (b) 15–20°C
    (c) 20–25°C
    (d) body temperature

12. The IDEAL method of removing contaminates from the surgical environment is:
    (a) dry vacuuming
    (b) sweeping
    (c) wet vacuuming
    (d) dusting

13. Which ONE of the following is NOT required to be **sterile** during a surgical scrub routine?
    (a) towels
    (b) scrubbing brush
    (c) gloves
    (d) scrub solution

14. Cleaning of **instruments** prior to sterilization:
    (a) is required to remove organic matter
    (b) should be done only with an ultrasonic cleaner
    (c) will damage delicate instruments
    (d) is not necessary if sterilization methods are good

15. The **ideal** time to damp dust the theatre area is:
    (a) first thing in the morning
    (b) immediately after a procedure
    (c) last thing at night
    (d) an hour prior to a procedure.

Organization of a theatre list

Consider the following procedures and organize them into clean, clean–contaminated, contaminated and infected categories. Now organize them into an operating list which will minimize the risk of contamination.

Number	Procedure
	Dog dentistry with extractions
	Bitch ovariohysterectomy
	Dog cruciate repair
	Enterotomy on a cat
	Flush rabbit abscess
	Cat dental (Felv) positive
	Aural ablation

Surgical instruments

Across
2. Scoop
5. Bowel clamps
6. Common scissor
7. Haemostats
10. Exposes site
11. Funny wire
12. Chuck
13. Scots needle holder

Down
1. Removing sutures
3. Gauges
4. Bone shaper
6. Can give you a sting
8. Rodent's mouth
9. Grasps tissue

Surgical instruments answers

¹P													
A				²C	U	³R	E	T	T	E			
Y	⁴O					R	O						
N	S		⁵D	O	Y	E	N	S		⁶M	A	Y	O
E	T					G				O			
⁷S	P	E	N	C	E	R	W	E	L	L	S		
	O				A		U			Q		⁹A	
¹⁰R	E	T	R	A	C	T	O	R		U		L	
	O				T		S		¹¹G	I	G	L	I
	M				O					T		I	
	E				O		¹²J	A	C	O	B	S	
					T					S			
		¹³M	C	P	H	A	I	L	S				

Answer key
Multiple choice

1. c	6. b	11. b
2. b	7. a	12. c
3. d	8. c	13. d
4. a	9. d	14. a
5. d	10. b	15. d

Number	Procedure
4	Dog dentistry with extractions
2	Bitch ovariohysterectomy
1	Dog cruciate repair
3	Enterotomy on a cat
7	Flush rabbit abscess
5	Cat dental (Felv) positive
6	Aural ablation

6
Selected reading

Cooper, B. (1997) *Veterinary Surgical Instruments: An Illustrated Guide.* Butterworth-Heinemann, Oxford (ISBN 0 7506 3613 0).

Edwards, B., Houlton, J. E. F. and Hickman, J. A. (1996) *An Atlas of Veterinary Surgery.* Blackwell Science, Oxford (ISBN 0 6320 3268 5).

Lane, D. R. and Cooper, B. (1999) *Veterinary Nursing.* Butterworth-Heinemann, Oxford (ISBN 0 7506 3999 7).

McBride, D. F. (1996) *Learning Veterinary Terminology.* Mosby, St Louis, MO (ISBN 0 8151 5960 9).

Tracy, D. L. (1999) *Small Animal Surgical Nursing.* Mosby, St Louis, MO (ISBN 1 5566 4503 1).

Index

Abdominal surgery, 29–43
cystotomy, 42–3
enterotomy/enterectomy,
38–9
laparotomy, 30–1
orchidectomy (castration),
36–7
ovariohysterectomy, 32–5
splenectomy, 40–1
Amputation kit, 64–5
Anaesthetic equipment, 21
Anal furunculosis, 67
Anal gland removal, 68–9
Approaches, surgical, 2
Artery forceps, 4
Aural surgery, 72–3

Biopsy, 78–9
Bitch spay, 32–3
Bone cutters, 6, 47
Bone rasps, 6
Bone-holding forceps, 6, 46,
47

Caesarean section, 33
Calculus removal, 83

Castration, 36–7
Conjunctival flap, 75
Cruciate repair kit, 60–1
Cryosurgical unit, 15–16,
17
Cryptorchidectomy, 37
Cyst removal, 81
Cystotomy, 42–3

Dentistry, 83–5
equipment, 5–6, 82–5
prophylactic, 83, 84–5
Diaphragm repair, 31
Diathermy unit, 15, 16
Digit amputation, 65
Disposables, 12–15, 22–3
Dissecting forceps, 4
Distichiasis, 75
Drains, surgical, 15
Drapes, 12, 13
Drills/drill bits, 6, 7

Ectropion, 75
Elevators, dental, 5
Endometritis, 33
Endoscopes, 16–17, 18

Enterectomy, 39
Enterotomy, 38–9
Entropion, 75
Enucleation, 75
Epiphyseal fracture repair,
  53
Excision arthroplasty,
  62–3

Forceps:
  artery, 4
  bone-holding, 6, 46, 47
  dissecting, 4
  tissue, 4
  tooth extraction, 5
Fracture fixation, 7, 49
  external fixation, 58–9
  rush pin repair, 50–1
  See also Orthopaedic
    equipment

Gastrotomy, 31
Gowns, 12, 13

Haematoma, 73
Health and safety, 28, 85
Hernia repair, 31
Hysterectomy, 33

Instrumentation, 22
  ophthalmic instruments, 5

Laparotomy, 30–1
Limb amputation, 65

Mandibular symphysis
  fracture repair, 53
Mastectomy, 31

Needles:
  holders, 4
  suture, 10–11
    atraumatic, 10
    cutting, 11
    eyed/traumatic, 10
    round-bodied, 10

Ophthalmic instruments, 5
Ophthalmic surgery, 74–5
Orchidectomy (castration),
  36–7
Orthopaedic equipment, 6–7,
  43–65
  amputation kit, 64–5
  cruciate repair kit, 60–1
  excision arthroplasty kit,
    62–3
  fracture fixation, 7, 49
    external fixation, 58–9
    rush pin repair, 50–1
  pinning equipment, 7,
    56–7
  plating equipment, 7, 54–5
  screws, 7
  wiring equipment, 7, 52–3
Ovariohysterectomy, 32–5
  bitch spay, 32–3
  cat spay, 34–5

Patella luxation repair, 61
Patient preparation, 26–7
Perineal surgery, 65–71

anal furunculosis, 67
anal gland removal, 68–9
urethotomy/urethostomy,
    70–1
Pinna repair, 73
Pinning equipment, 7,
    56–7
Plating equipment, 7, 54–5
Prefixes, 1
Probes, dental, 6

Retractors, 5
    orthopaedic, 6
Rongeurs, 6
Rupture repair, 31
Rush pin fracture repair,
    50 1

Safety, 28, 85
Scalers, 5
Scalpel:
    blade handle, 3
    blades, 3
Scissors, 4
Screws, 7
Scrotal ablation, 37
Spay:
    bitch, 32 3
    cat, 34–5
Splenectomy, 40 1
Sterilization equipment, 22
Suction unit, 17, 18
Suffixes, 1–2
Surgical personnel:
    health and safety, 28, 85
    preparation, 24–6
    surgical scrub, 24–6

Surgical procedures, 29–85
    abdominal surgery, 29–43
        cystotomy, 42–3
        enterotomy/
            enterectomy, 38–9
        laparotomy, 30–1
        orchidectomy
            (castration), 36–7
        ovariohysterectomy,
            32–5
        splenectomy, 40–1
    aural surgery, 72–3
    biopsy, 78–9
    environment preparation,
        23
    equipment preparation,
        21–3
    ophthalmic surgery, 74–5
    orthopaedic surgery,
        43–65
        amputation, 64–5
        cruciate repair, 60–1
        excision arthroplasty,
            62–3
        fracture fixation, 7, 49,
            58–9
        pinning equipment, 7,
            56–7
        plating equipment, 7,
            54–5
        rush pin fracture repair,
            60–1
        wiring equipment, 7,
            52 3
    patient preparation, 26–7
    perineal surgery, 65–71
        anal furunculosis, 67
        anal gland removal,
            68–9

urethotomy/
    urethostomy, 70–1
surgical approaches, 2
thyroidectomy, 76–7
Suture materials, 7–11, 80–1
    alternatives to, 10
    classification of, 8–9
        absorbable, 9
        non-absorbable, 9
    ideal characteristics of, 8
    needles, 10–11
Swabs, 12–13

Tail amputation, 65
Tendon repair, 53
Terminology, 1–2
Theatre:
    environment preparation,
        23
    equipment preparation, 22
    requirements, 17–20

Thyroidectomy, 76–7
Tissue forceps, 4
Tooth extraction forceps,
    5
Towel clips, 4
Trochleoplasty, 61
Tumour removal, 31, 67, 73,
    81
    eyelid, 75

Urethostomy, 70–1
Urethotomy, 71

Visceral clamps, 5

Wire cutters/twisters, 6,
    52–3
Wound classification, 2

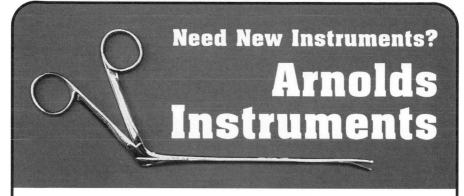

Need New Instruments?
Arnolds Instruments

We offer General Surgical, Ophthalmic, Orthopaedic, Tungsten Carbide and External Fixation

For your catalogue and demonstration
contact Arnolds Veterinary Products Ltd

01743 441632

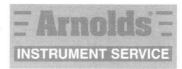

With Arnolds quick and convenient Instrument Service, you no longer have to reject your old instruments, you can rejuvenate them.

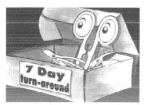

It's also quick! In seven days your instruments are returned to you - re-tightened, re-groved, re-sharpened, re-finished, repaired (with a six month gaurantee) or replaced (with your approval).

So take advantage of Arnolds' Instrument Service today

Contact Arnolds to receive your freepost box 01743 441632

Arnolds®

www.arnolds.co.uk

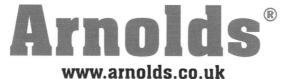

For further info please contact Arnolds Veterinary Products Ltd, Cartmel Drive, Harlescott, Shrewsbury, SY1 3TB Tel +44 (0)1743 441632 Fax +44 (0)1743 462111